My Fruit
ADVENTURES

A Journal for Food Discovery and
Exploration Using Your 5 Senses

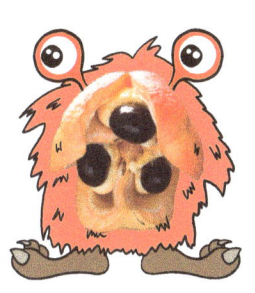
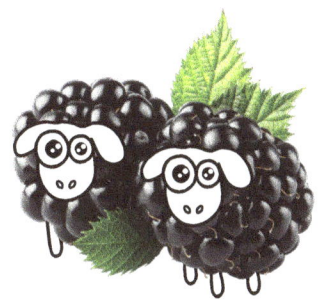
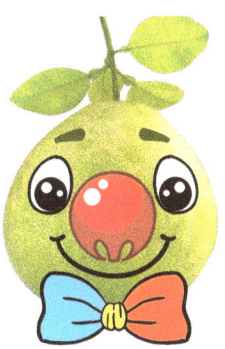

This journal belongs to:

> PULL UP A CHAIR.
> TAKE A TASTE.
> COME JOIN US.
> LIFE IS SO ENDLESSLY
> DELICIOUS.
>
> Ruth Reichl

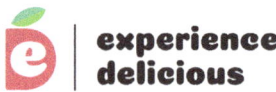

Experience Delicious LLC

All Rights Reserved. This book or any portion thereof may not be reproduced or used in any manner whatsoever without the express written permission of the publisher except for the use of brief quotations in a book review.

Copyright 2019 Experience Delicious, LLC.
ISBN: 978-1-947001-20-6
www.experiencedeliciousnow.com

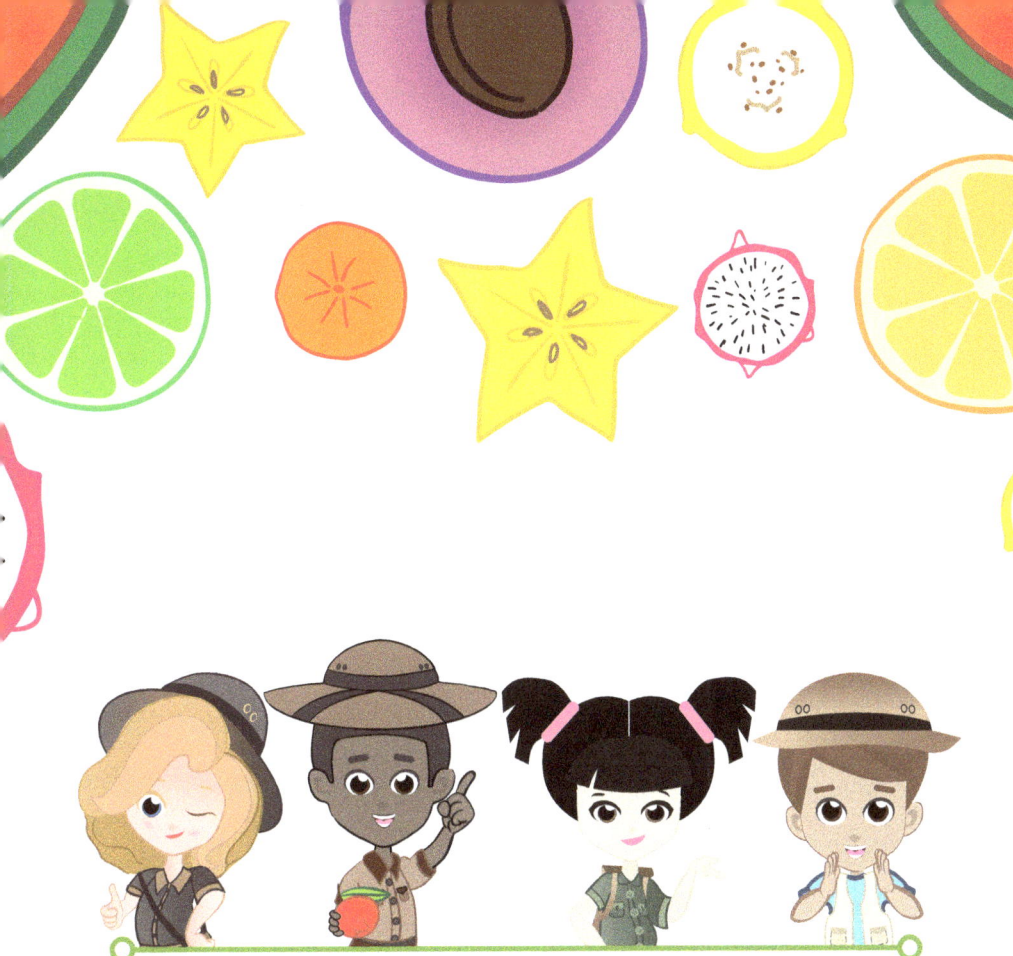

Welcome Food Explorer!

It's time to experiment with fruit using your five senses! Conduct your own taste-tests with new fruits or old favorites prepared in different ways. Try different varieties of the same fruit side by side. Learn how to use descriptive words while discovering flavors and textures. Get ready to learn more about YOUR fruit preferences!

This journal is your personal fruit exploration log. It is designed to track your adventures with fruit and provide a space for you to write and talk about what you like and don't like about them.

Don't forget to include your parents, caregivers, and friends on your search for delicious and ask for help when needed! Now put on your Food Explorer hat, pick a fruit to try, grab your crayons or colored pencils, and dig in!

Let's start by drawing your favorite fruit!

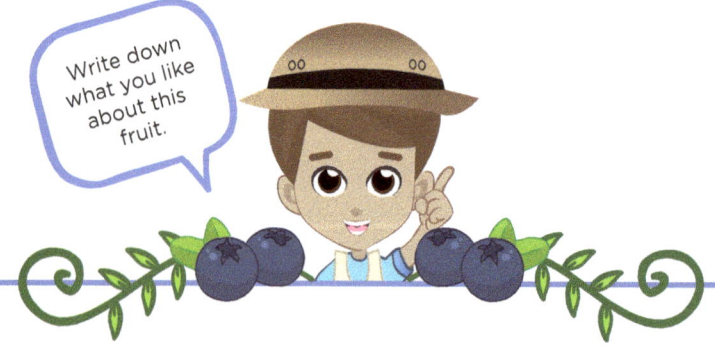

Write down what you like about this fruit.

Next, draw your least favorite fruit.

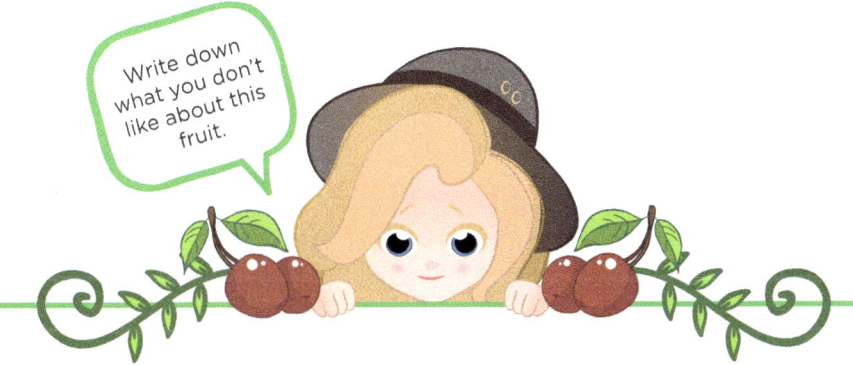

Using Your 5 Senses

Have you ever explored fruit?

Think about what fruit you like to eat.
What do you like about them?
How do you like to eat them?

There are so many wonderful and delicious ways to prepare fruit! Do you like fruit raw, squeezed into juice, or baked into dessert? Have you ever tried a fruit grilled, dried, or made into a jam?

Exploring fruits with our 5 senses is fun and can help us discover and engage with what we eat.

When you taste-test a fruit, take a moment to observe how it looks, how it smells, how it sounds, how it feels in your mouth, and how it tastes using your 5 senses.

Get creative, it's okay to play with your food!

5 Senses

Can you describe a fruit? Each preparation method can change the experience. We can use our 5 senses to discover things we never knew we liked about a food!

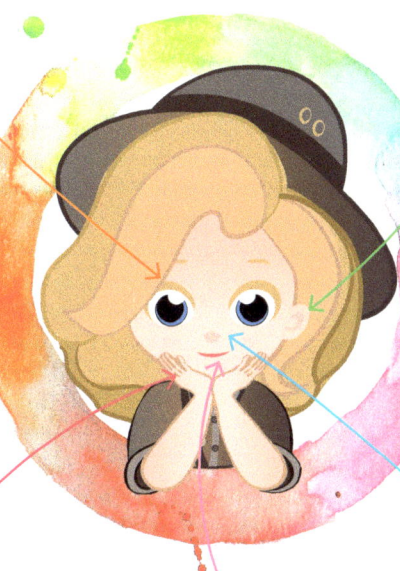

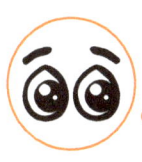

See

Take a closer look at the fruit. What colors and textures do you SEE? Does it remind you of anything?

Hear

What sound do you HEAR when you run your fingers over the skin? Is it silent or does it make a sound? Now take a bite. Did you HEAR anything? Keep chewing. Are there any sounds? Is each bite a loud crunch or a quiet chew?

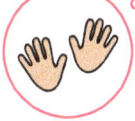

Feel

How does the skin FEEL in your hands? Is the texture rough, smooth, or silky? What about when you peel the skin? What does the texture FEEL like in your hands or when you take a bite? Is it firm, sticky, or mushy? Is each bite soft and tender? Try it raw or prepared!

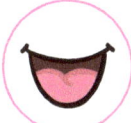

Taste

How does it TASTE? What is the flavor like? Can you describe it? Is it sweet or sour? Does it have a flavor at all? Does it TASTE different when it is raw than when it is prepared another way? Which do you like better and why?

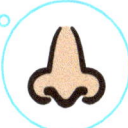

Smell

Have you ever sniffed your fruit? That might sound silly, but SMELLING food is a big part of tasting! Hold a piece of fruit up to your nose and take a good whiff. What does it SMELL like? Does it SMELL floral, sweet, or candy-like? Does it have a scent at all?

100 Descriptive Words

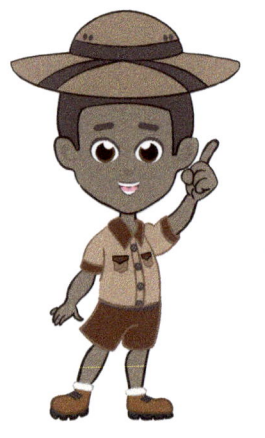

Descriptive words help us identify unique qualities about foods and explain what we like or dislike about them.

When you sit down for a meal or snack, take a moment to think about how it looks, how it smells, how it sounds, how it feels in your mouth, and how it tastes using your 5 senses. It's like your very own experiment every time you eat!

When a food feels, looks, smells, or tastes similar to another food you can say it is "like" another food or add a "y" at the end of the word. Such as butter-like, celery-like, or honey-like and citrusy, lemony, or watery.

WORD	DESCRIPTION	SENSE(S)
Acidic	bitter, sharp, sour	Taste
Ambrosial	delicious, fragrant, sweet	Smell · Taste
Aroma; Aromatic	scent, smell, odor	Smell
Astringent	mouth-puckering, sharp	Taste
Bitter	acidic, harsh, sharp, sour	Taste
Bland	flavorless, mild	Taste
Bright	acidic, sharp, tart, giving out or reflecting light, shiny appearance	See · Taste
Burnt	charred, crunchy, overcooked	Feel · See · Smell · Taste · Hear
Buttery	creamy, rich, smooth, velvety, feels similar to butter	Feel · Taste
Chewy	leathery, sticky, tough	Feel
Complex	multiple aromas, flavors, or textures	Feel · Smell · Taste
Creamy	smooth, velvety	Feel
Crisp(y)	crunchy, firm, snappy	Feel · Hear
Crunchy	brittle, crisp, loud	Feel · Hear
Delicate	fine texture, light or subtle taste, tender	Feel · Taste
Dense	compact, heavy, thick	Feel
Distinctive	unlike other flavors or textures, unique qualities	Feel · Taste
Dry	free of liquid or moisture	Feel · See · Taste
Earthy	feels, smells, or tastes similar to soil	Feel · Smell · Taste
Exotic	different, unusual, unfamiliar	See · Taste
Fibrous	stringy, thick, tough	Feel
Firm	hard, solid, stiff	Feel

WORD	DESCRIPTION	SENSE(S)
Flavorful; Flavorsome	having a lot of flavor	Taste
Flesh(y)	pulpy, soft, thick	Feel
Floral; Flowery	smells or tastes similar to a flower	Smell · Taste
Fluffy	airy, light	Feel · See · Taste
Fragrant	sweet smell or scent, perfumed	Smell
Fresh	new, peak of ripeness, unspoiled	Feel · See · Smell · Taste
Fruity	varies and can mean citrusy, sweet, or tangy	Smell · Taste
Fuzzy	fibrous, furry, or hairy coating	Feel · See
Gelatinous	gluey, gummy, jelly-like, sticky	Feel · See · Taste
Glossy	glazed, polished, shiny	See
Grainy	coarse, granular, gritty	Feel · See
Gritty	coarse, grainy, granular, rough	Feel · See · Taste
Hard	firm, solid	Feel
Herbal	smells or tastes similar to an herb	Smell · Taste
Honeyed	feels, looks, smells, or tastes similar to honey	Feel · See · Smell · Taste
Intense	sharp, strong, powerful	Smell · Taste
Juicy	full of juice or liquid, succulent	Feel · Hear · See
Knobby	lumpy surface, rounded	See
Light	contains air, does not make you feel full quickly, lacks a strong color, smell, or taste	Feel · See · Smell · Taste
Mealy	crumbly, dry, grainy	Feel · See
Meaty	dense, thick, taste or texture similar to meat	Feel · Taste
Melting	dissolve, liquify	Feel · See · Smell · Taste
Metallic	looks, smells, or tastes similar to metal	See · Smell · Taste
Mild	bland, free of a strong smell or taste	Smell · Taste
Milky	creamy, feels, looks, smells, or tastes similar to milk	Feel · See · Taste
Moist	slightly damp or wet	Feel · See
Mushy	may feel spoiled, soft, wet	Feel
Musky	fragrant odor, natural scent, pungent	Smell · Taste
Nutty	tastes similar to nuts	Taste
Odor	aroma, musk, scent	Smell
Peppery	hot, pungent, spicy, smells or tastes similar to pepper	Smell · Taste
Piney	looks, smells, or tastes similar to pine	See · Smell · Taste
Piquant	flavorful, tangy, zesty, pungent in smell or taste	Smell · Taste
Plump	fleshy, full, round	Feel · See
Pulpy	fibrous, fleshy, soft	Feel · See
Pungent	bitter, hot, peppery, sharp, powerful smell or taste	Smell · Taste
Refreshing	cool, fresh, or different	Feel · Smell · Taste
Rich	creamy, dense, fatty, full-flavored, heavy, strong and pleasant smell or taste	Feel · Taste · Smell
Robust	hearty, powerful, rich	Feel · See · Smell · Taste

WORD	DESCRIPTION	SENSE(S)
Rotten	bad, moldy, spoiled	Taste · See · Smell
Rough	bumpy, textured, uneven surface	Taste · See · Feel
Rubbery	elastic, flexible, tough, similar to rubber	Feel · See
Savory	delicious smell or taste, having a salty or spicy quality without sweetness, well-seasoned	Taste · Smell
Seeded	having seeds	Feel · Hear · See
Shrivel	shrink, wither, wrinkle	Feel · See
Silky	glossy, smooth, soft, similar to silk	Feel · See
Skunky	aromatic, smells or tastes spoiled	Smell · Taste
Slimy	gooey, slippery, wet, feels similar to slime	Feel · See
Smooth	even, flat, uniform consistency	Feel · See
Soft	smooth, easy to press	Feel · See
Sour	acidic, bitter, tart, similar to lemon or vinegar	Feel · Smell · Taste
Spicy	aromatic, hot, peppery, pungent, strongly flavored	Smell · Taste
Spongy	airy, light, soft, feels similar to a sponge	Feel · See
Starchy	feels or tastes similar to other high starch foods such as potatoes or rice	Feel · Taste
Sticky	glue-like, syrupy, tacky, viscous	Feel · See
Stinky	unpleasant smell	Smell
Subtle	delicate, faint, light	Smell · Taste
Succulent	delicious, juicy, yummy	Feel · See · Smell · Taste
Sugary	sweet, honeyed, similar to sugar	Feel · See · Smell · Taste
Sweet	smells or tastes similar to sugar or honey	Smell · Taste
Sweet-Sour	both sweet and sour	Feel · Smell · Taste
Sweet-Tart	both sweet and tart	Feel · Smell · Taste
Syrupy	luscious, moist, thick or sweet similar to syrup	Feel · See · Smell · Taste
Tacky	gluey, gummy, sticky	Feel · Hear · See ·
Tang(y)	aromatic, flavorful, sharp, strong	Smell · Taste
Tart	acidic, sharp, sour	Feel · Taste
Tasteless	without flavor	Taste
Tender	delicate, soft	Feel
Textured	touchable or visual quality or characteristic	Feel · See
Tough	dense, fibrous, hard	Feel
Tropical	aromas and flavor similar to those found in the tropics	Smell · Taste
Velvety	delicate, smooth, soft	Feel
Vibrant	bright, colorful, zesty, zippy	See · Smell · Taste
Watery	feels, looks, or tastes similar to water	Feel · See · Taste
Waxy	shiny, sticky, similar feel and look to wax	Feel · See
Wrinkly	bumps, creases, or folds on a surface	See
Zesty	pungent, seasoned, sharp, spicy, tart	Smell · Taste
Zippy	fresh, invigorating	Taste

Let's practice!
Use 5 words to describe this fruit.

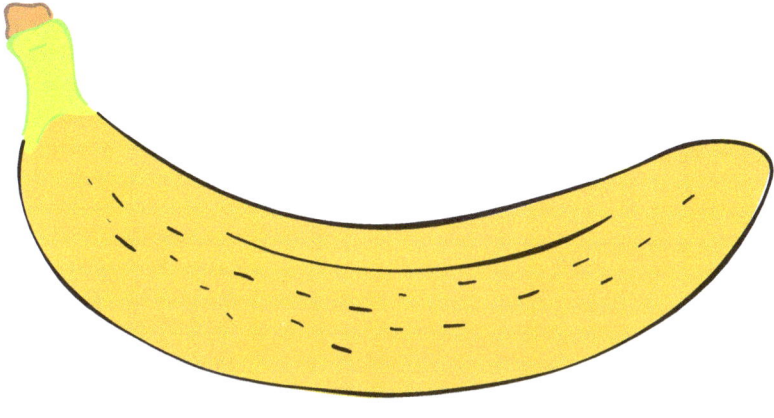

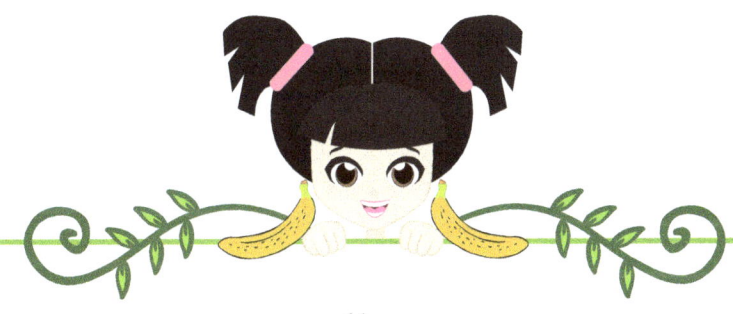

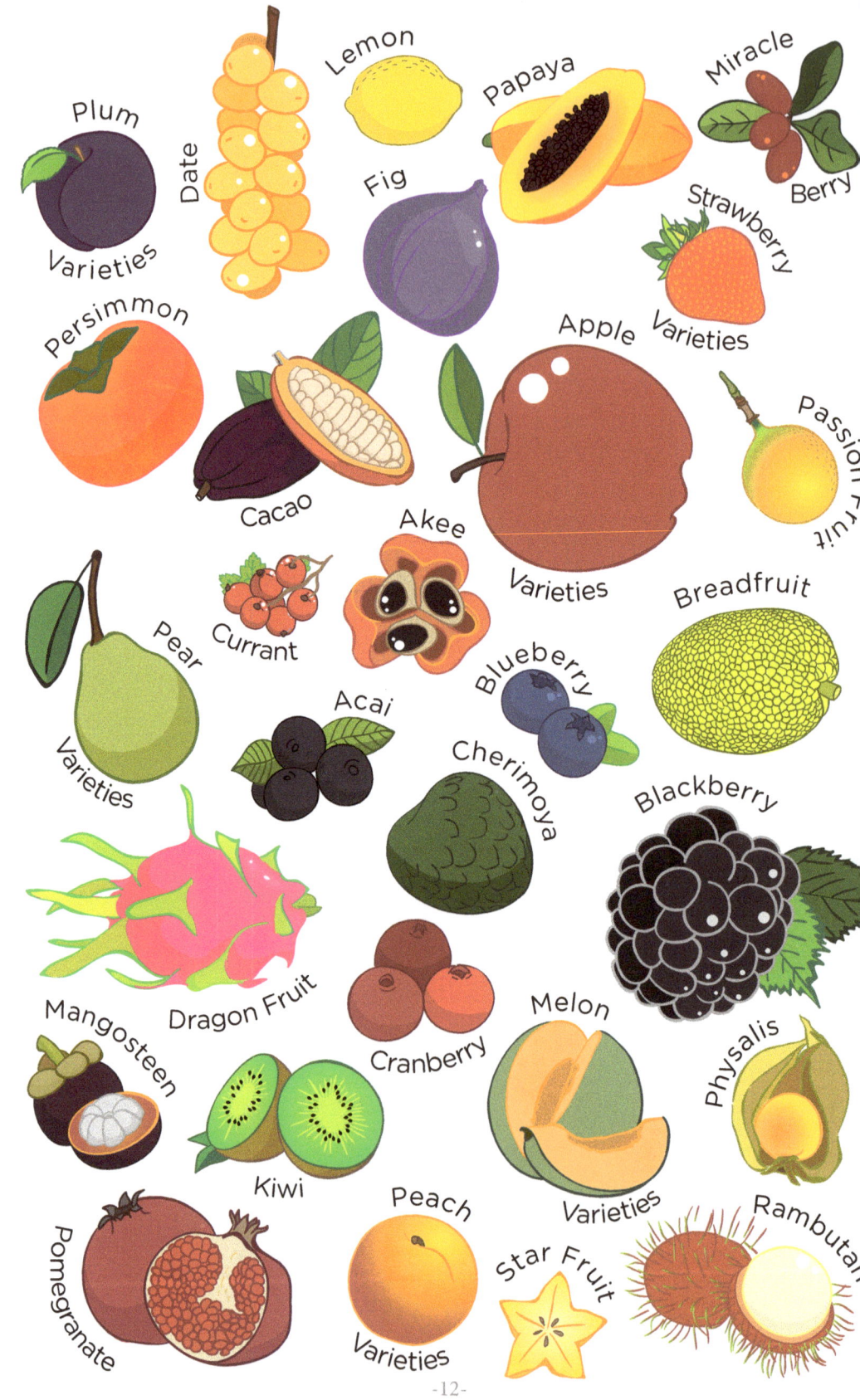

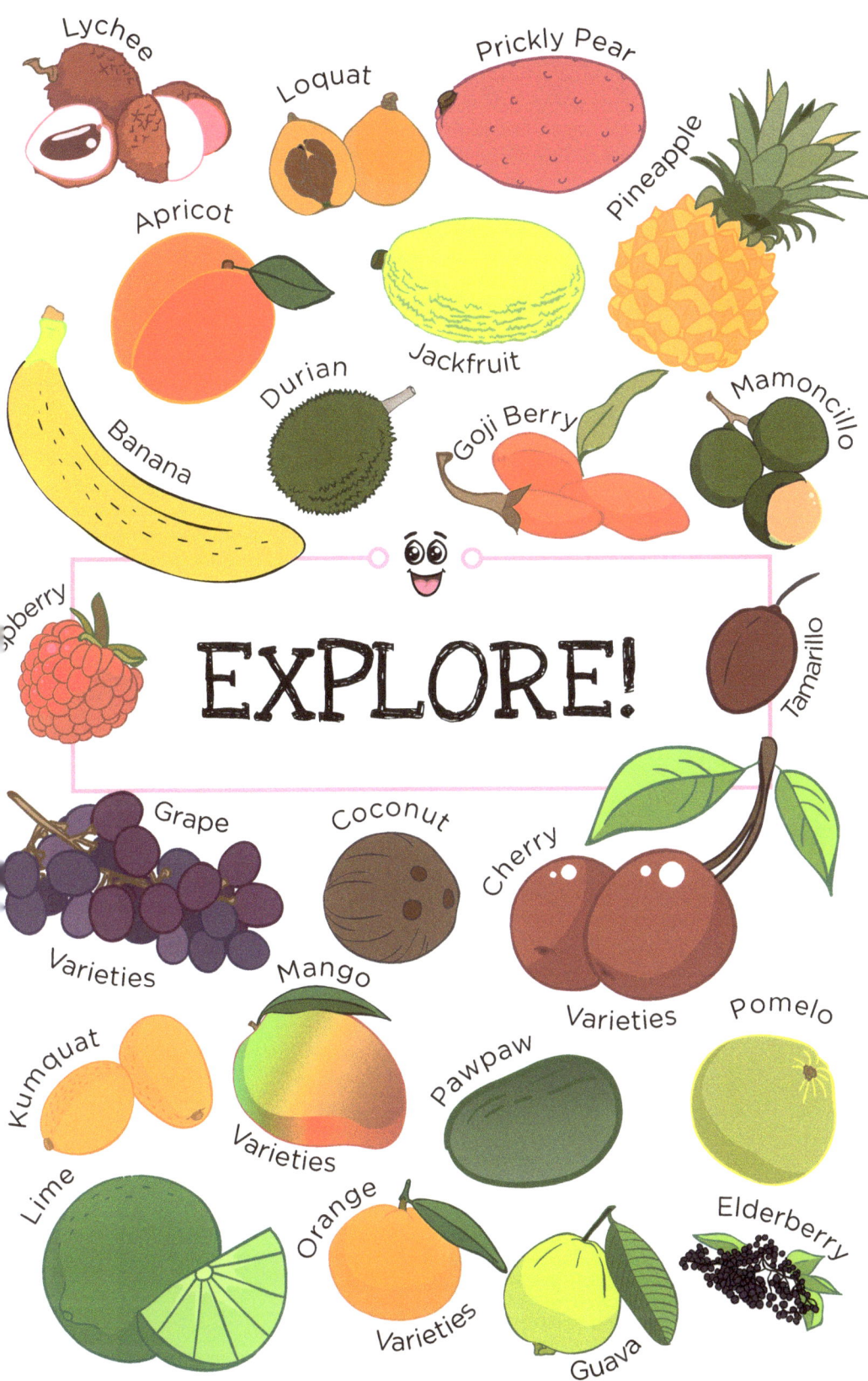

Fruit Name _____ **Date** _____

Preparation Method _____

Did you like this fruit?

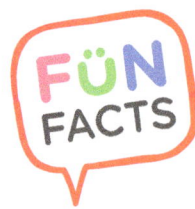

Most apples look and feel waxy because the skin produces a protective covering of wax that keeps them moist and firm (think crunchy!). This slows down how long it takes to get moldy. Sometimes additional wax is added to increase how long appples can be stored.

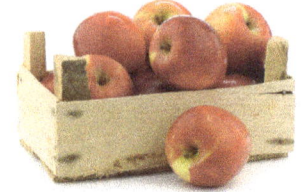

Fruit Name _____ **Date** _____

Preparation Method _____

_____

_____

_____

_____

_____

_____

_____

_____

_____

_____

_____

_____

_____

_____

Did you like this fruit?

Apple Varieties

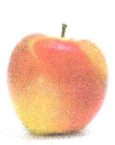   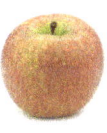   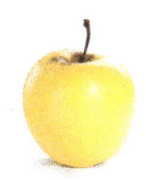   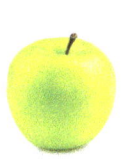   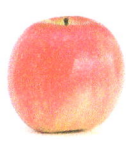   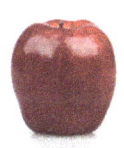

Braeburn   Fuji   Golden Delicious   Granny Smith   Pink Lady   Red Delicious

Fruit Name _____ **Date** _____

Preparation Method _____

_____

_____

_____

_____

_____

Did you like this fruit?

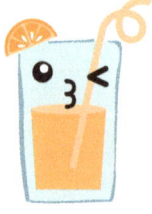

Cooking Method

Juices and smoothies transform fruits and vegetables into a liquid that is ready to drink. Juicing removes the liquid from a food and smoothies blend food into a liquid.

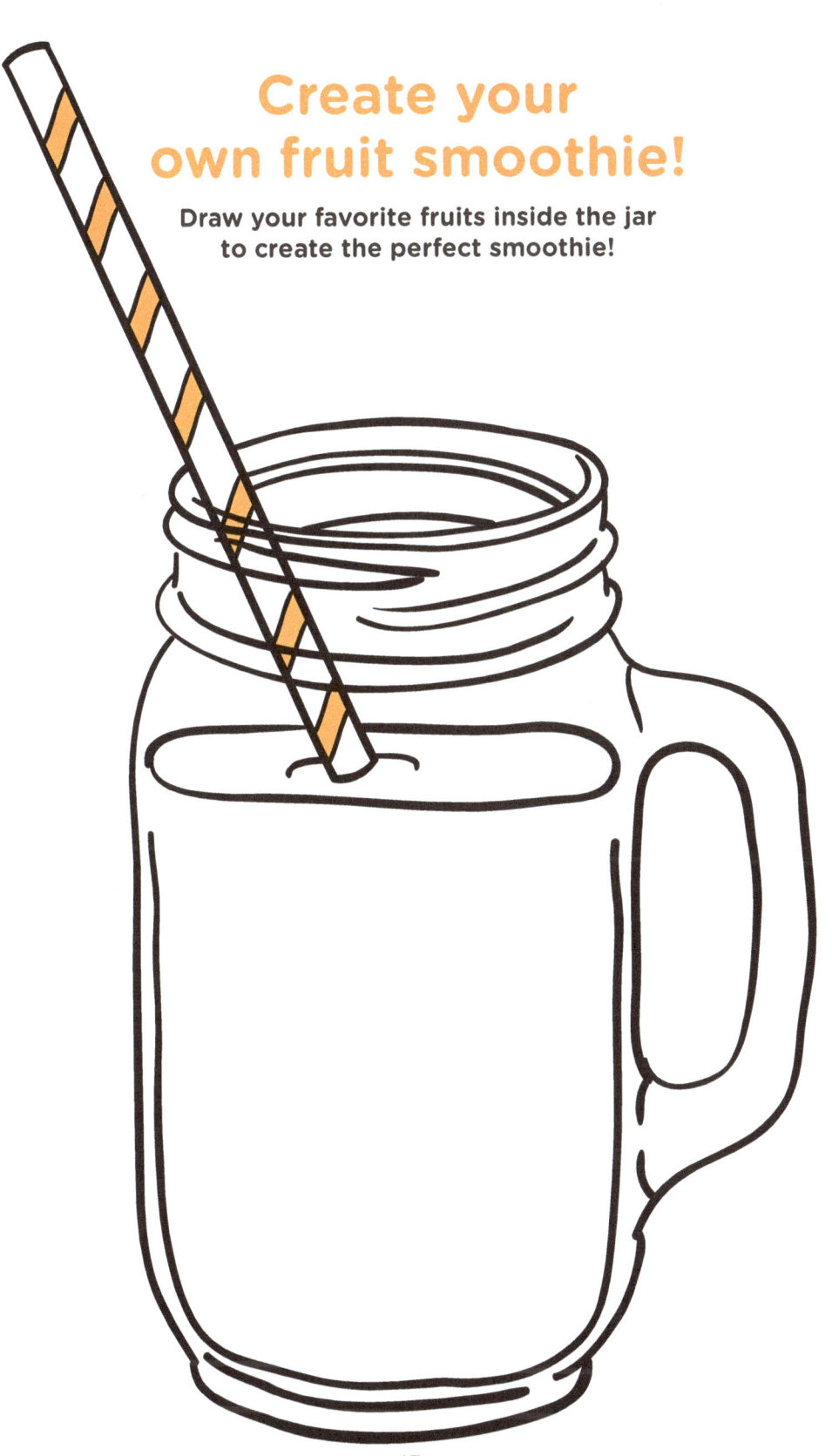

Fruit Name _____   **Date** _____

Preparation Method _____

_____

_____

_____

_____

_____

_____

_____

_____

_____

_____

Did you like this fruit?

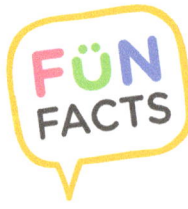

A sweet, aromatic variety of lemon, the Meyer lemon, is thought to be a natural hybrid between a lemon and a mandarin orange. Meyer lemons are small, rounded, and yellow to orange in color. They are great candied, in sauces, and juiced for lemonade.

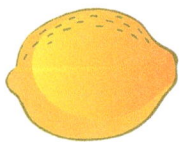

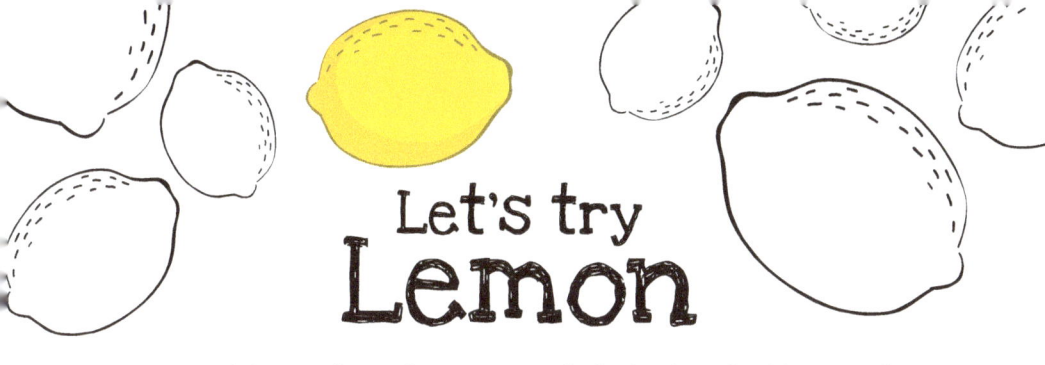

Let's try Lemon

Pick golden yellow, firm, smooth fruit that feel heavy for their size. Lemons should be free of dark or soft spots.

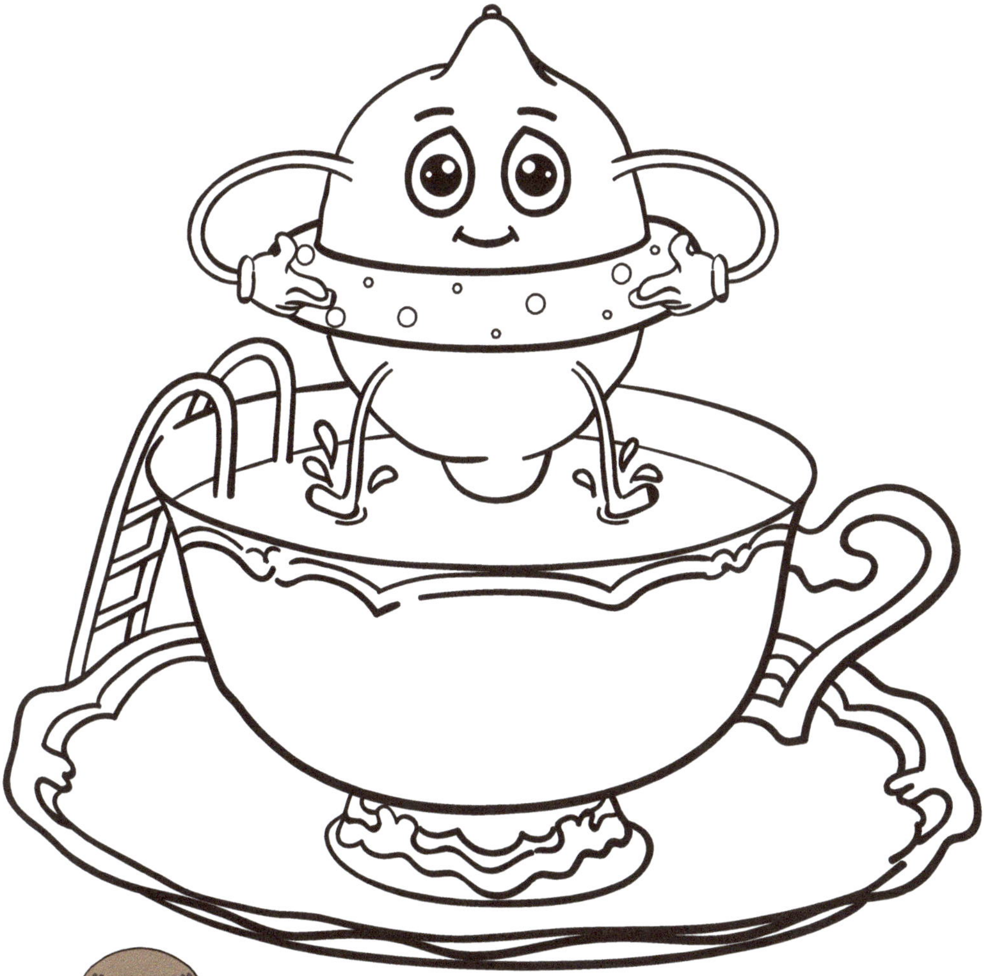

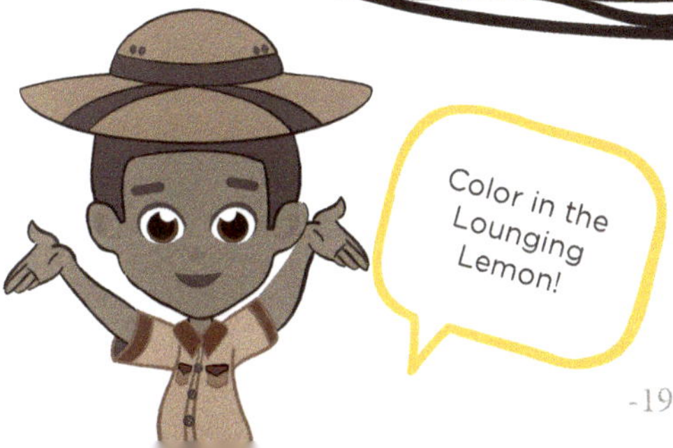

Color in the Lounging Lemon!

Fruit Name _____   **Date** _____

Preparation Method _____

_____
_____
_____
_____
_____
_____
_____
_____
_____
_____
_____
_____
_____
_____
_____

Did you like this fruit?

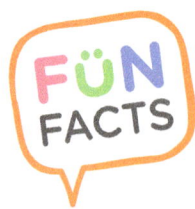 In some parts of the world there are festivals and celebrations when goji berries are harvested each year.

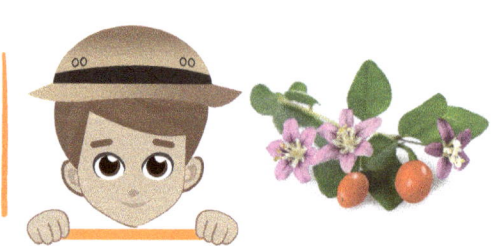

Fruit Name ⎯⎯⎯⎯⎯⎯⎯⎯⎯⎯⎯⎯⎯⎯⎯⎯⎯⎯⎯ **Date** ⎯⎯⎯⎯⎯⎯⎯

Preparation Method ⎯⎯⎯⎯⎯⎯⎯⎯⎯⎯⎯⎯⎯⎯⎯⎯⎯⎯⎯⎯⎯⎯⎯⎯⎯⎯

Did you like this fruit?

Draw what you're tasting!

Fruit Name _____   **Date** _____

Preparation Method _____

_____
_____
_____
_____
_____
_____
_____
_____
_____
_____
_____
_____
_____
_____
_____

Did you like this fruit?

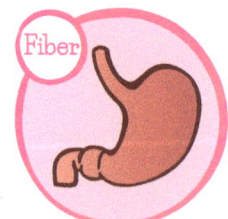

Good for My Body Nutrient

Fiber helps keep your heart healthy, your insides clean by moving food through your digestive system, and makes your tummy feel full. Digestion is how your body gets nutrients and energy from the food you eat.

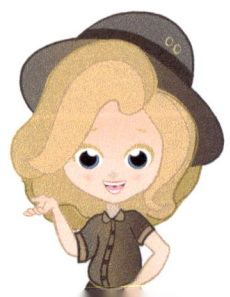

Fruit Name _____   **Date** _____

Preparation Method _____

Did you like this fruit?

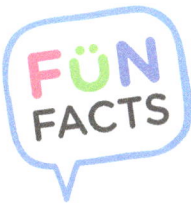 One of a giraffe's favorite food is wild apricot trees! They eat the leaves and the fruit.

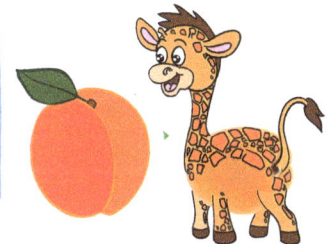

Fruit Name _____ **Date** _____

Preparation Method _____

_____
_____
_____

_____
_____
_____

_____
_____
_____

_____
_____
_____

_____
_____

Did you like this fruit?

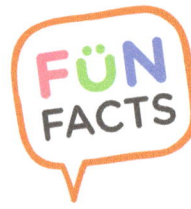

Oranges have many varieties and hybrids. In fact, mandarin is the group name for a type of orange with a thin, loose peel. Tangerines are a type of mandarin. All tangerines are mandarin oranges, but not all mandarin oranges are tangerines! There are so many varieties of citrus fruit that originate from the orange.

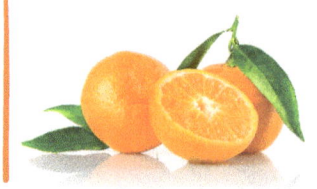

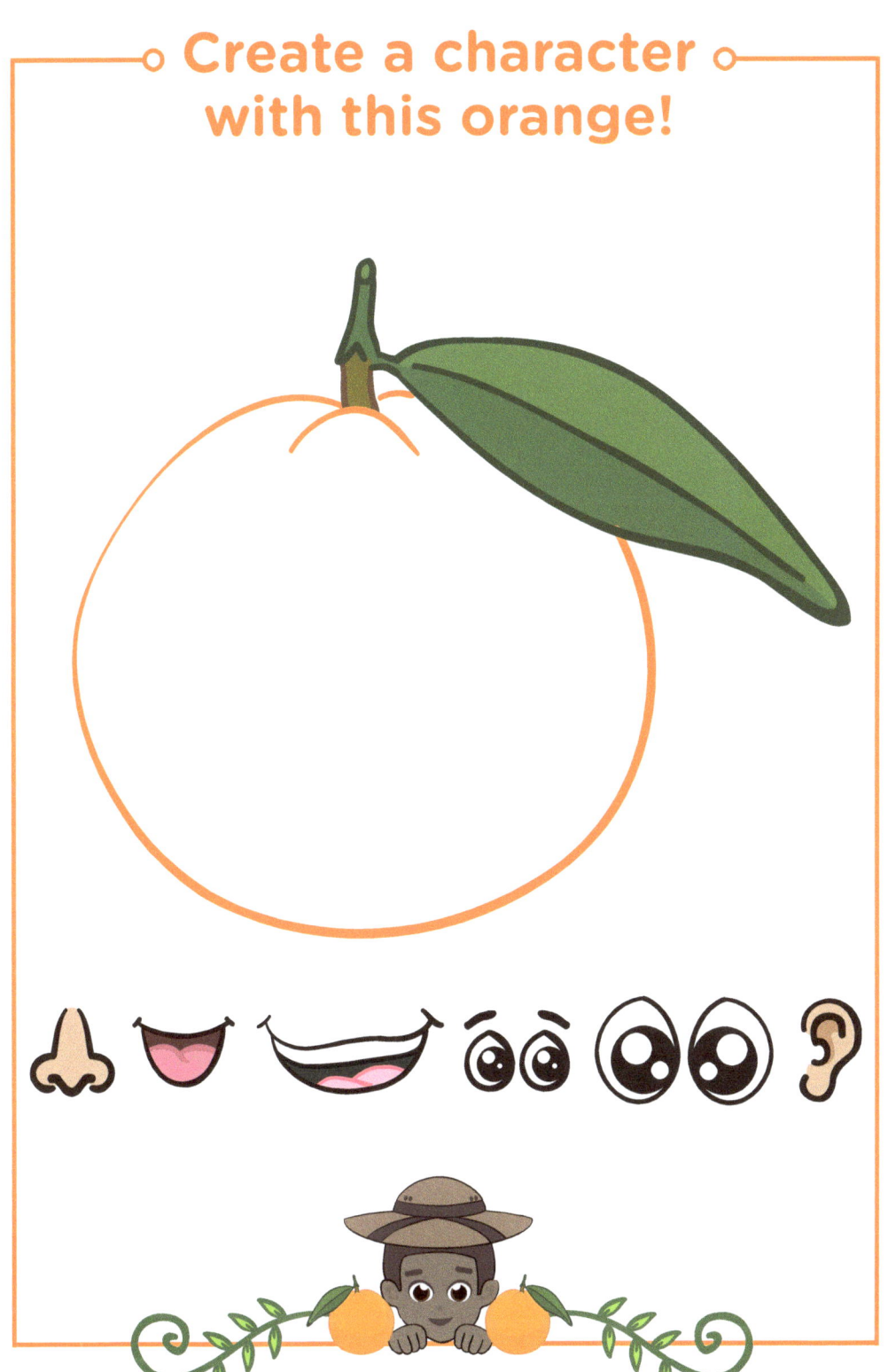

Fruit Name _____ **Date** _____

Preparation Method _____

_____

_____

_____

_____

_____

_____

_____

_____

_____

Did you like this fruit?

DID YOU KNOW?

Coconuts are considered a tropical drift seed because they float and can survive years at sea. The ocean is a way for coconuts to spread their seeds and grow coconut palm trees in new locations.

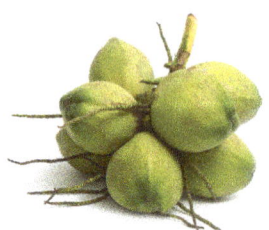

Fruit Name _____   Date _____

Preparation Method _____

Did you like this fruit?

Draw what you're tasting!

Let's compare the same fruit prepared two ways!

Fruit Name _____ **Date** _____

Preparation Method _____

_____
_____
_____
_____
_____
_____
_____
_____
_____
_____

Did you like this fruit?

Which cooking method did you like better?

_____
_____

Let's compare the same fruit prepared two ways!

Fruit Name _____ **Date** _____

Preparation Method _____

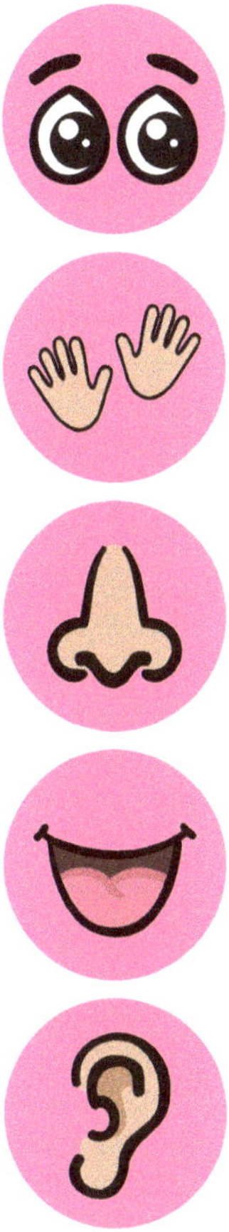

_____

_____

_____

_____

_____

Did you like this fruit?

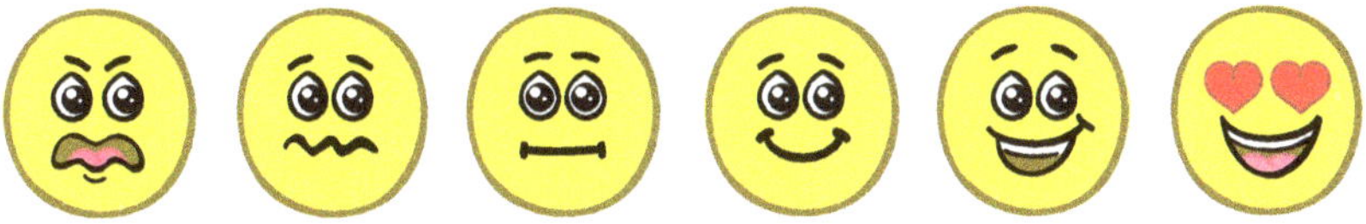

Why did you like it?

_____

Fruit Name _____   **Date** _____

Preparation Method _____

_____

_____

_____

_____

_____

Did you like this fruit?

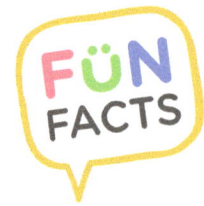

The flesh on some fruits such as apples and bananas turn brown when exposed to oxygen or air. To prevent browning, brush or dip fruit slices in lemon, lime, pineapple, or orange juice. The vitamin C in these juices helps protect fruit from the air.

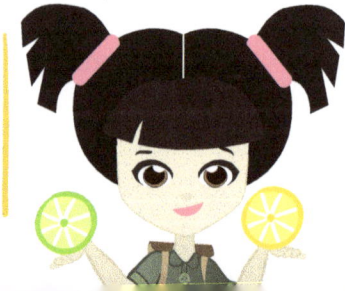

Fruit Name _____   **Date** _____

Preparation Method _____

Did you like this fruit?

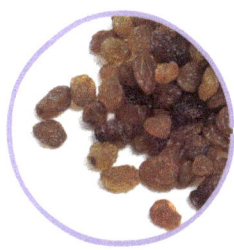

Dried grapes are called raisins. In ancient Rome, raisins were highly valued and used as a form of currency or money.

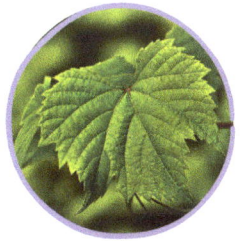

Young, tender grape leaves are edible and can be stuffed with a variety of savory fillings including rice, meat, and cheese.

Fruit Name _____   **Date** _____

Preparation Method _____

_____

_____

_____

_____

_____

_____

_____

Did you like this fruit?

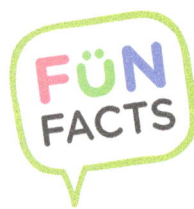

The seeds of mamoncillo can be roasted and eaten like chestnuts or ground into a flour and used as a substitute for cassava flour.

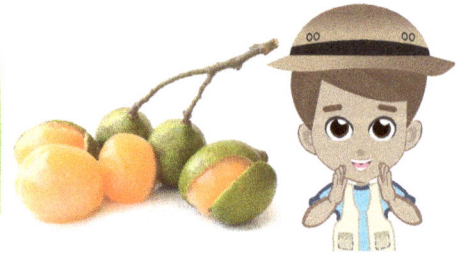

Why do you eat fruit?

How do you choose what new fruit you will try?

Fruit Name _____ **Date** _____

Preparation Method _____

_____

_____

_____

_____

_____

Did you like this fruit?

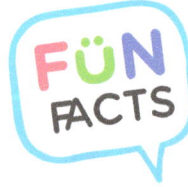 Ripe fruit is ready to be eaten. Want to ripen a fruit fast? Place fruit in a brown paper bag. This will trap a gas called ethylene that is naturally released during ripening and helps to soften fruit.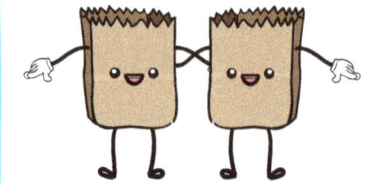

Fruit Name _____   **Date** _____

Preparation Method _____

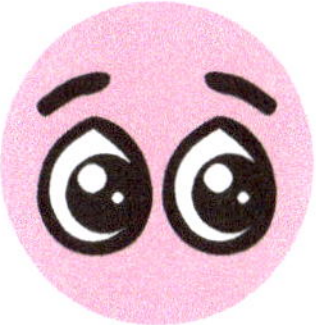

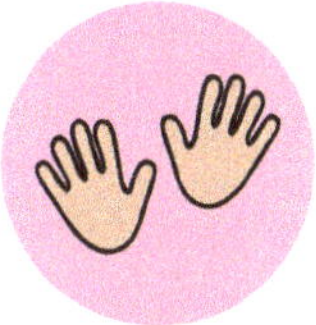

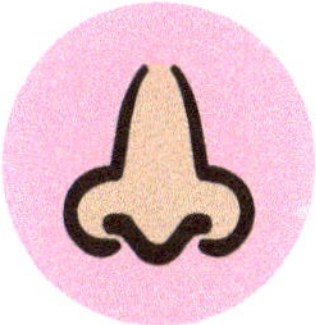

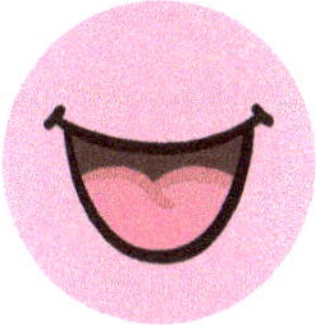

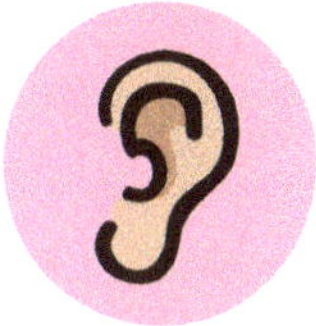

_____
_____
_____
_____
_____
_____
_____
_____
_____
_____

Did you like this fruit?

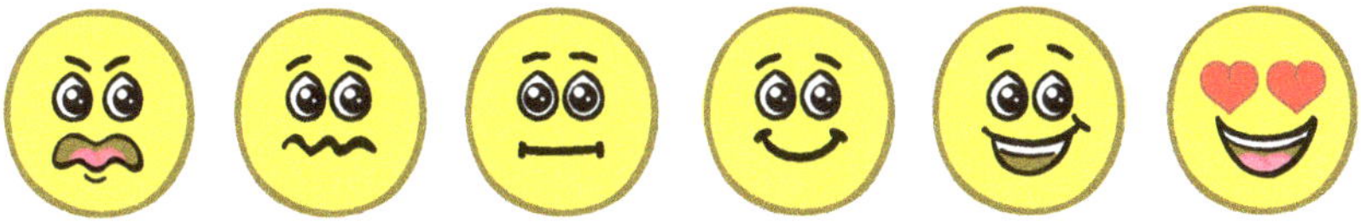

Tasting Notes

_____
_____
_____

Fruit Name _____   **Date** _____

Preparation Method _____

_____

_____

_____

_____

_____

Did you like this fruit?

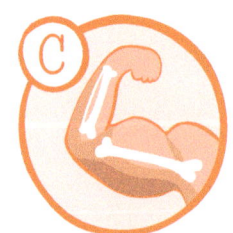

Good for My Body Nutrient

Vitamin C promotes strong muscles and bones so you can be active and play your favorite sports. Vitamin C also supports healthy skin, teeth, brain cells, and helps heal cuts when you get a scrape.

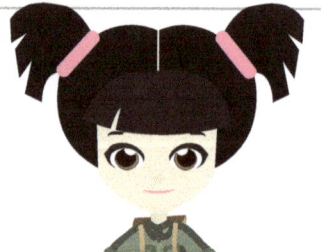

**Create a new fruit!
Draw what it looks like and describe
its flavors and textures.**

Fruit Name _____   **Date** _____

Preparation Method _____

_____
_____

_____
_____

_____
_____

_____
_____

_____
_____

Did you like this fruit?

DID YOU KNOW?

Miracle berry makes sour foods taste sweet and changes the perceived sweetness of foods. Miracle berry is often eaten for fun at tasting parties where participants eat a berry and then taste a variety of tart and astringent foods. It transforms:

lemon ⟶ lemonade
sour candy ⟶ sweet candy

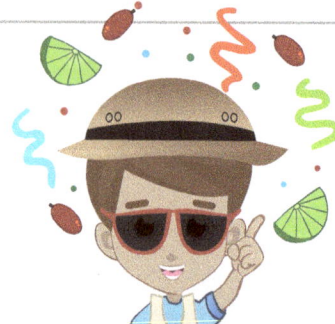

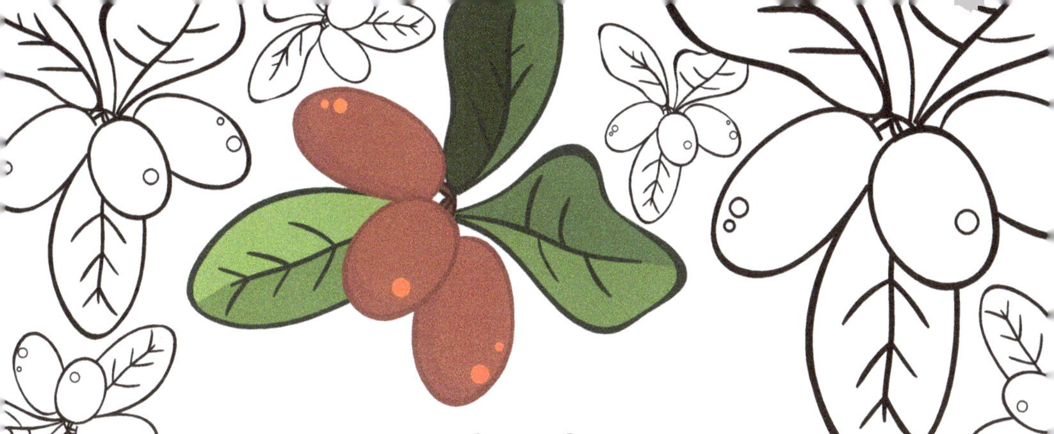

Let's try
Miracle Berry

Miracle berry are typically sold frozen, freeze-dried, dehydrated, or in tablet form because they spoil very quickly. For fresh miracle berry, pick bright red, firm fruit with a smooth surface.

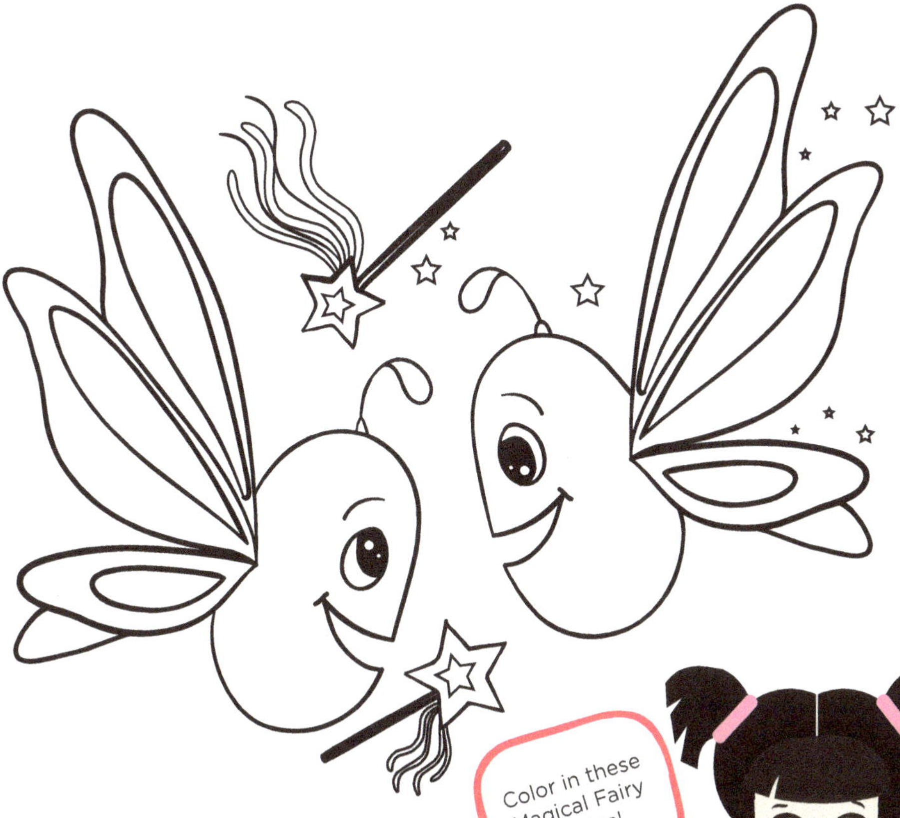

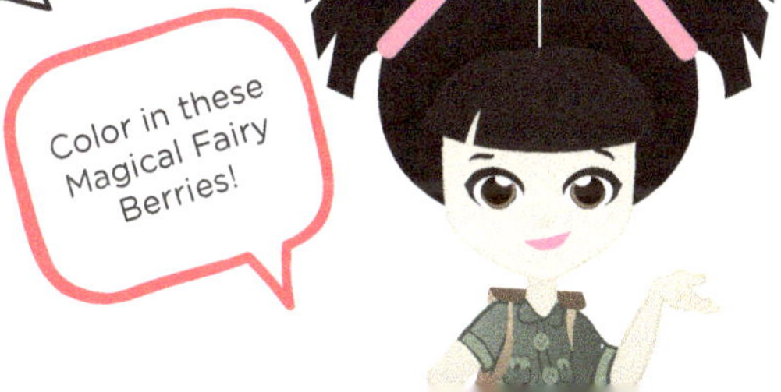

Color in these Magical Fairy Berries!

Fruit Name _____ **Date** _____

Preparation Method _____

_____

_____

_____

_____

_____

_____

_____

_____

_____

_____

_____

Did you like this fruit?

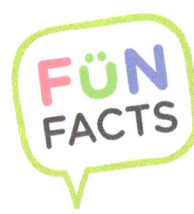 British sailors in the 1800's were given a daily allowance of limes to eat for long voyages across the ocean to prevent scurvy. Scurvy is a sickness as a result of not eating enough Vitamin C. Scurvy causes teeth to loosen and skin to bruise easily, or turn black and blue.

Fruit Name _____   **Date** _____

Preparation Method _____

Did you like this fruit?

Draw what you're tasting!

Fruit Name _____ **Date** _____

Preparation Method _____

_____

_____

_____

_____

_____

Did you like this fruit?

DID YOU KNOW?

The two most common varieties of kumquats are meiwa and nagami. Meiwa are more rounded in shape and have a sweeter flavor than the oval-shaped nagami.

Kumquats are about the size of your thumb.

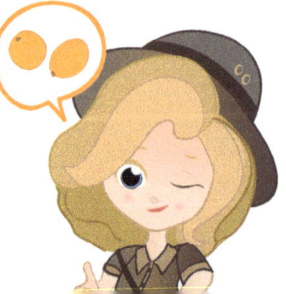

Fruit Name _____   **Date** _____

Preparation Method _____

_____

_____

_____

_____

_____

Did you like this fruit?

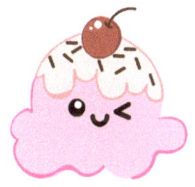

Cooking Method

Desserts are sweet foods such as cakes, cookies, ice cream, pies, and pudding. Desserts are typically served at the end of a meal.

Let's compare the same fruit prepared two ways!

Fruit Name _____   **Date** _____

Preparation Method _____

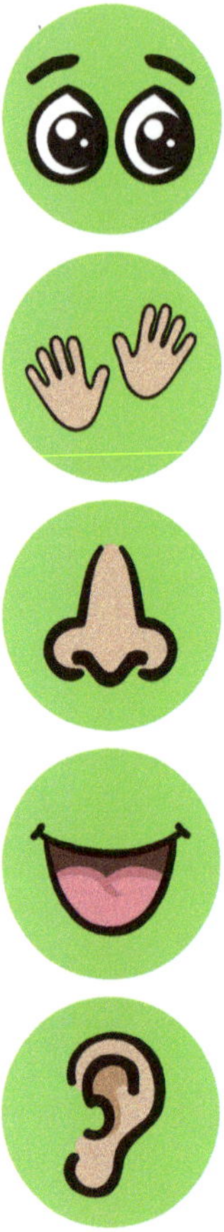

Did you like this fruit?

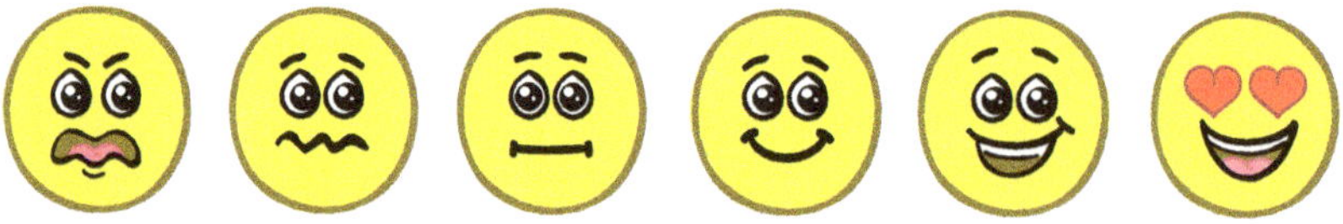

Which cooking method did you like better?

_____

Let's compare the same fruit prepared two ways!

Fruit Name _____ **Date** _____

Preparation Method _____

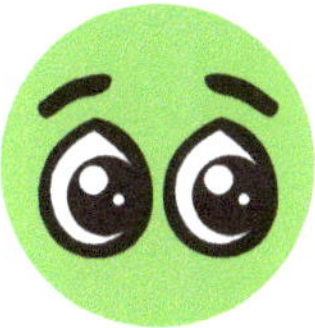

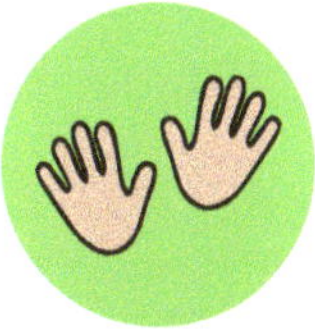

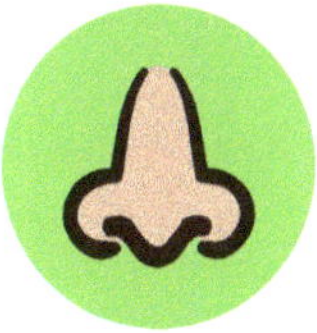

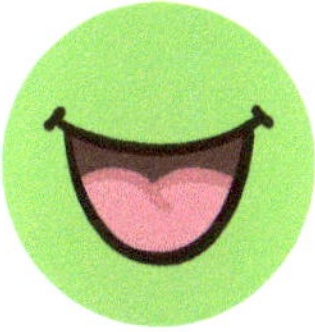

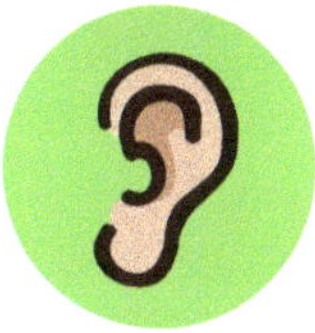

Did you like this fruit?

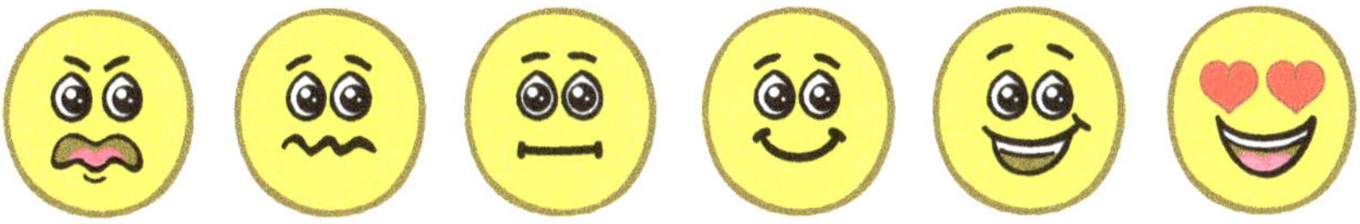

Why did you like it?

Fruit Name _____ **Date** _____

Preparation Method _____

_____

_____

_____

_____

_____

Did you like this fruit?

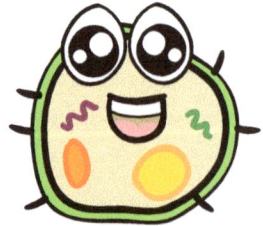

DID YOU KNOW?

When pears fully ripen on the tree, they can become gritty because of something called stone cells. Stone cells are the same material that make cherry stones and walnuts shells hard. Pears harvested before they ripen typically have a more even, smooth texture.

Fruit Name _____ **Date** _____

Preparation Method _____

_____

_____

_____

_____

_____

Did you like this fruit?

Pear Varieties

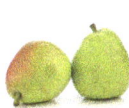 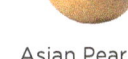 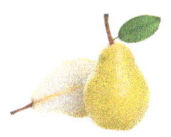 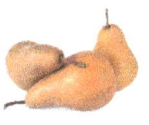 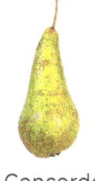 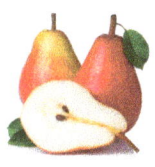

Anjou   Asian Pear   Barlett   Bosc   Concorde   Forelle

Fruit Name _____ **Date** _____

Preparation Method _____

Did you like this fruit?

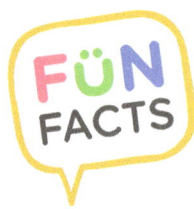

Physalis are surrounded by a papery, light brown husk called the calyx that looks like a lantern. Peel back the husk to reveal the fruit!

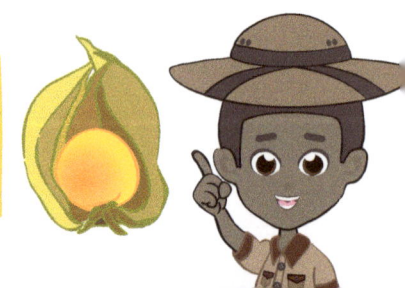

Let's try fruit varieties!

Fruit Name _____

Draw the variety and describe its flavor using descriptive words.

Variety: **Variety:**   **Variety:**

Fruit Name _____

Draw the variety and describe its flavor using descriptive words.

Variety: **Variety:**   **Variety:**

Fruit Name _____ **Date** _____

Preparation Method _____

_____
_____

_____
_____

_____
_____

_____
_____

_____
_____

Did you like this fruit?

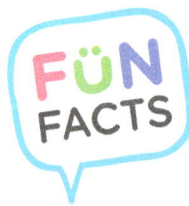

Native Americans in North America introduced blueberries to the Pilgrims as "star berries" because the blossom end of each berry looks like a star. The star, or calyx, forms a perfect, five-pointed star.

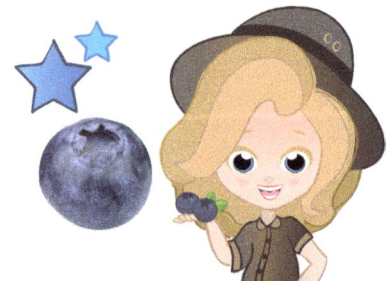

Fruit Name _____ **Date** _____

Preparation Method _____

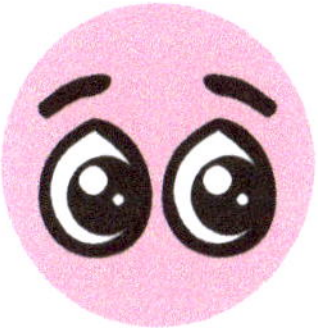

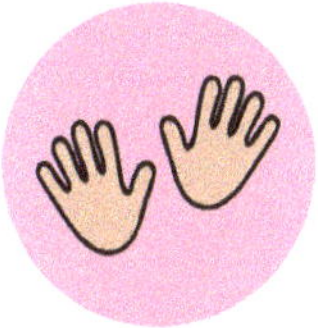

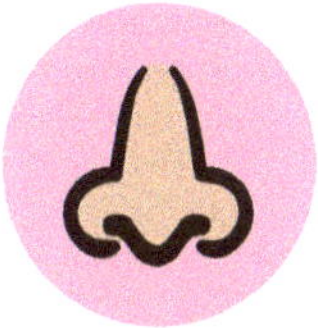

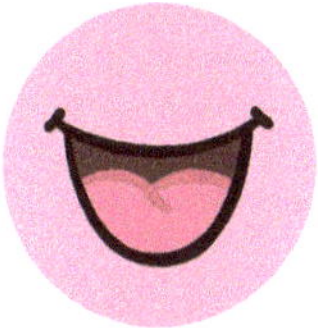

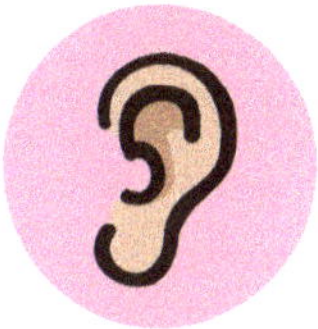

_____

_____

_____

_____

_____

_____

_____

_____

_____

_____

_____

Did you like this fruit?

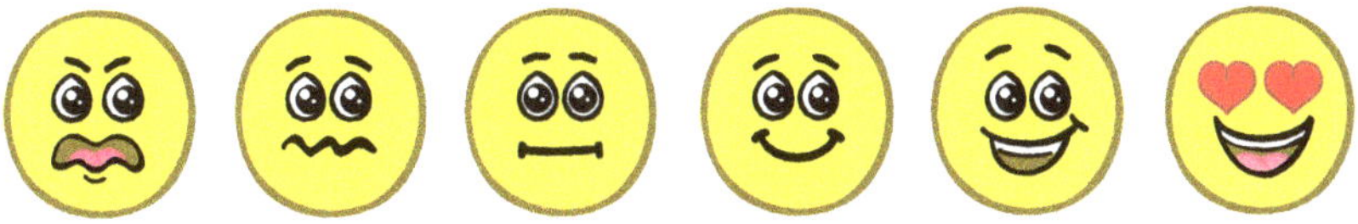

Tasting Notes

_____

_____

_____

Fruit Name _____   **Date** _____

Preparation Method _____

_____
_____
_____
_____
_____
_____
_____
_____
_____
_____
_____
_____

Did you like this fruit?

DID YOU KNOW?

There are over 1,200 known varieties of watermelon! The thick, hard rinds of watermelon vary from dark to pale green, solid to striped, and round to oval in shape.

Pick a fruit and draw what it looks like on the inside.

Fruit Name _____ **Date** _____

Preparation Method _____

_____

_____

_____

_____

_____

_____

_____

_____

Did you like this fruit?

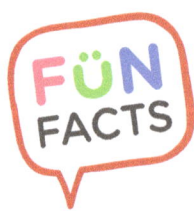 The red jewels inside pomegranates are called arils. Arils are the sweet-tart juice that surrounds the small white crunchy seeds inside the fruit. You can try the arils whole or spit out the seeds.

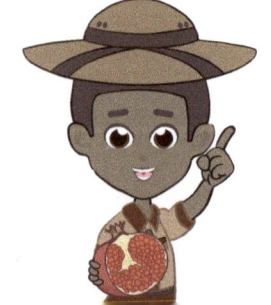

Fruit Name _____   **Date** _____

Preparation Method _____

(eyes) _____
_____

(hands) _____
_____

(nose) _____
_____

(mouth) _____
_____

(ear) _____
_____

Did you like this fruit?

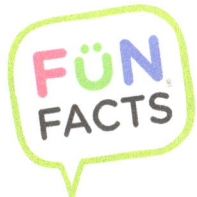

If you slice a star fruit in cross-sections, the pieces are shaped like a 5, 6, or 7-pointed star!

Fruit Name _____ **Date** _____

Preparation Method _____

_____
_____
_____
_____
_____
_____
_____
_____
_____
_____
_____
_____

Did you like this fruit?

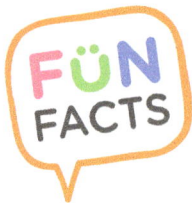 Strawberries are unlike other fruit because they bear their seeds on the outside of the fruit rather than the inside. Each strawberry has around 200 seeds! Can you count them all?

Fruit Name _____ **Date** _____

Preparation Method _____

_____
_____
_____
_____

_____
_____
_____
_____

_____
_____
_____
_____

_____
_____
_____
_____

_____
_____
_____
_____

Did you like this fruit?

Draw what you're tasting!

Fruit Name _____   **Date** _____

Preparation Method _____

Did you like this fruit?

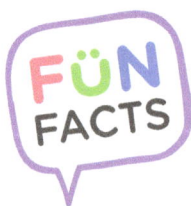

Figs are considered the sweetest fruit. They have a natural sugar content of 55%! Have you ever tried a fig for dessert?

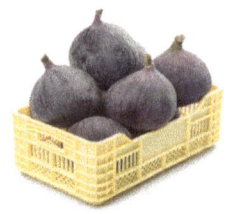

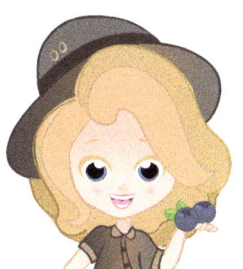

What's your favorite way to prepare fruit?

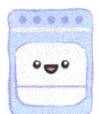
Bake

Baked Goods

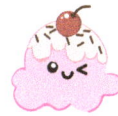
Dessert

Dried

Garnish

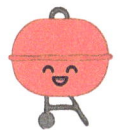
Grill

Jam

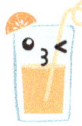
Juice

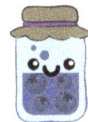
Pickle

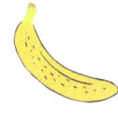
Raw

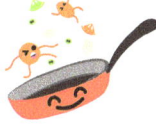
Sauté

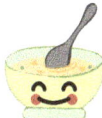
Soup

Tasting Notes

What's your favorite fruit recipe?

Fruit Name _____   **Date** _____

Preparation Method _____

_____

_____

_____

_____

_____

Did you like this fruit?

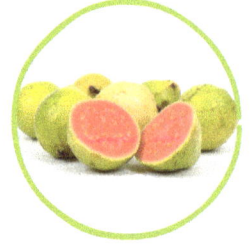

DID YOU KNOW?

There are over 100 different varieties of guavas with varying sizes, colors, textures, and flavors.

Fruit Name _____   **Date** _____

Preparation Method _____

Did you like this fruit?

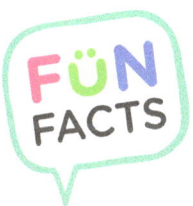

Jackfruit win the size contest. They are the largest fruit grown on trees with some weighing over 100 pounds!

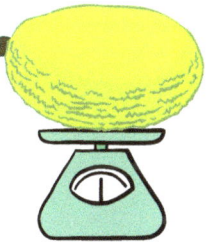

Fruit Name _____ **Date** _____

Preparation Method _____

Did you like this fruit?

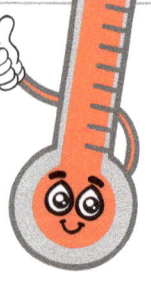

DID YOU KNOW?

Temperature is a measurement that indicates how hot or cold something is and can be measured using a thermometer in degrees Fahrenheit or degrees Celsius.

Plant your favorite fruit here!

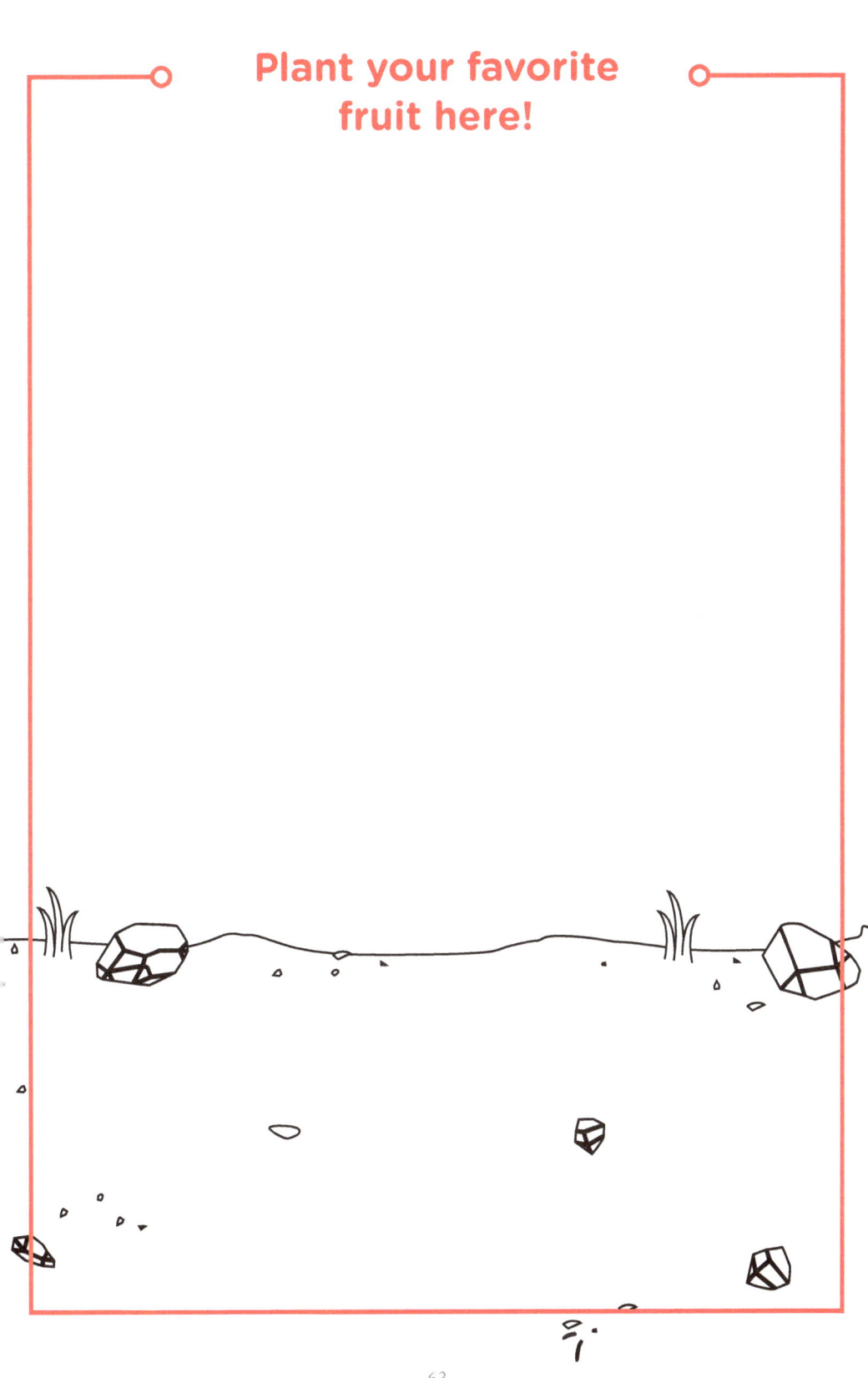

Fruit Name _____ **Date** _____

Preparation Method _____

_____
_____

_____
_____

_____
_____

_____
_____

_____
_____

Did you like this fruit?

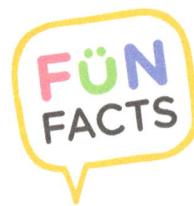

A single pineapple plant only produces one pineapple each fruiting season. Once picked, pineapples do not continue to ripen or sweeten, they only get juicier.

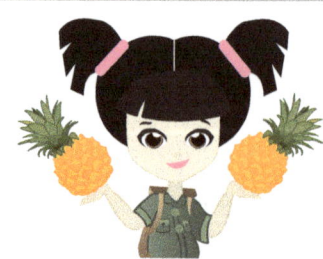

Let's try Pineapple

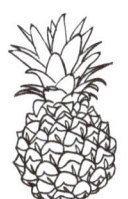 

Pick green to yellow-gold, plump, firm fruit that feel heavy for their size and have a sweet aroma. Pineapples should be free of dry looking skin, dirty leaves, soft spots, or a fermented, sour aroma.

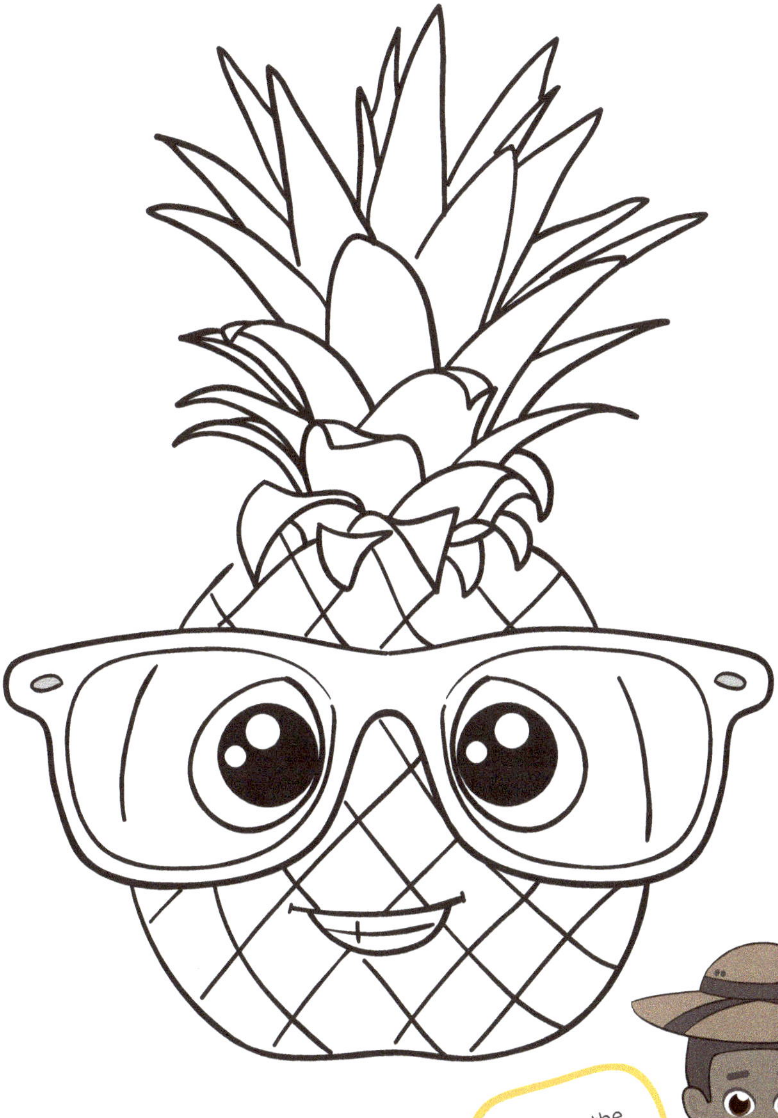

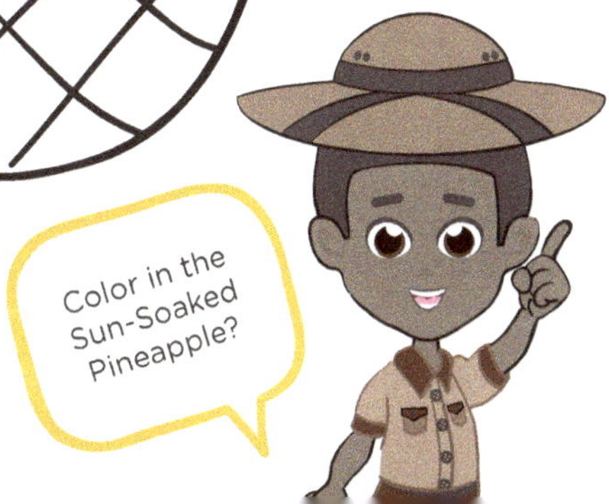

Color in the Sun-Soaked Pineapple?

Fruit Name _____ **Date** _____

Preparation Method _____

Did you like this fruit?

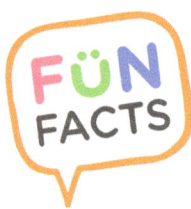 The sweet flesh of the lychee fruit is translucent. This means that light can pass through the fruit but you cannot see what is on the other side.

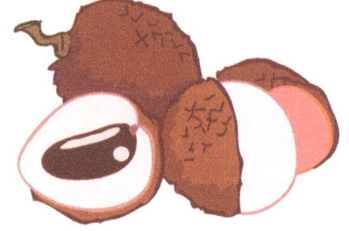

Fruit Name _____ **Date** _____

Preparation Method _____

Did you like this fruit?

 Some fruit plants need lots of sunlight while others grow in the shade.

 Many fruits thrive or grow in warm weather and others flourish or grow in cold weather.

Fruit Name _____   **Date** _____

Preparation Method _____

Did you like this fruit?

DID YOU KNOW?

Researchers believe that the strong scent of the durian developed over time to attract animals to eat the fruit and spread its seeds.

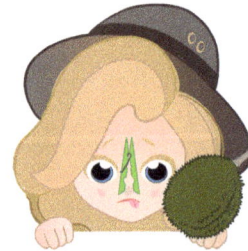
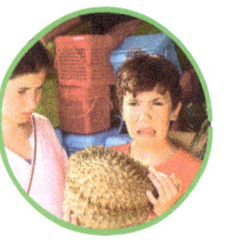

Fruit Name _____   **Date** _____

Preparation Method _____

Did you like this fruit?

Draw what you're tasting!

Fruit Name _____   **Date** _____

Preparation Method _____

_____
_____

_____
_____

_____
_____

_____
_____

_____
_____

Did you like this fruit?

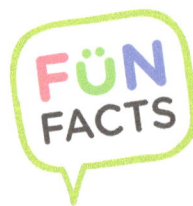

Persimmon trees are often used as edible landscaping. Edible landscaping is a gardening technique that uses fruit and vegetable plants and herbs rather than lawns or decorative trees and flowers. This promotes a cycle of growth and harvest rather than maintenance and results in food to eat.

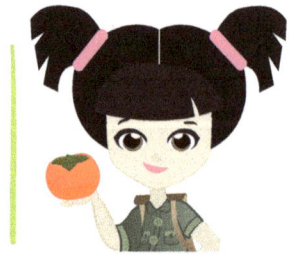

Let's try fruit varieties!

Fruit Name _____

Draw the variety and describe its flavor using descriptive words.

Variety: **Variety:**   **Variety:**

Fruit Name _____

Draw the variety and describe its flavor using descriptive words.

Variety: **Variety:**   **Variety:**

Fruit Name _____   **Date** _____

Preparation Method _____

Did you like this fruit?

DID YOU KNOW?

Have you ever seen a vegetable scrubber? It can help you clean the skin of vegetables by removing dirt and sand.

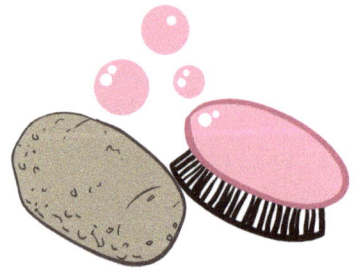

Fruit Name _____   **Date** _____

Preparation Method _____

_____

_____

_____

_____

_____

_____

Did you like this fruit?

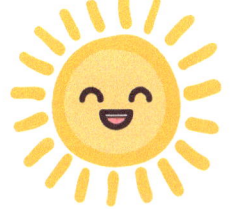

Cooking Method

Dried foods are a preparation method that removes water or juice through sun drying, dry heat, or dehydrators.

Fruit Name _____ **Date** _____

Preparation Method _____

_____

_____

_____

_____

_____

Did you like this fruit?

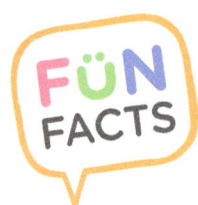 An individual banana is called a finger and a bunch of bananas are called a hand.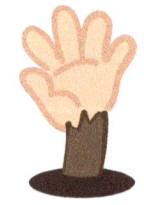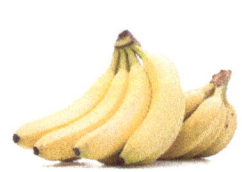

Open your fridge and draw the fruit you see!

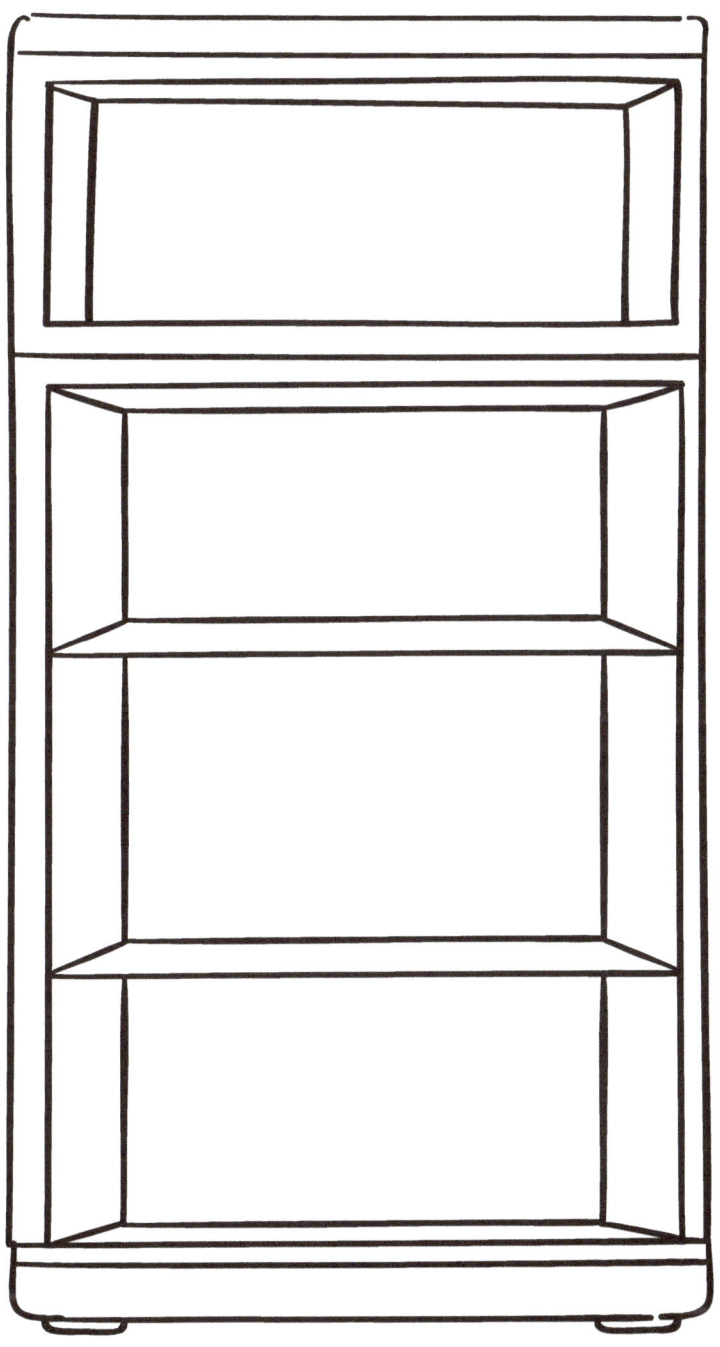

Fruit Name _____   **Date** _____

Preparation Method _____

Did you like this fruit?

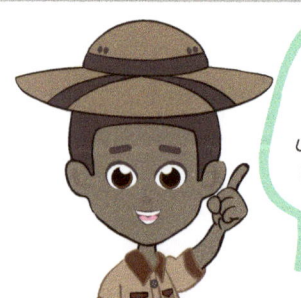

Always ask an adult to help you in the kitchen, especially when using knives or heat to prepare foods!

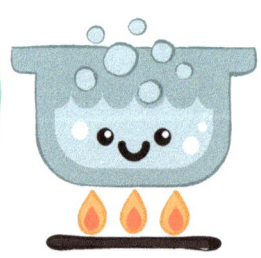

Fruit Name _____ **Date** _____

Preparation Method _____

Did you like this fruit?

Tasting Notes

Fruit Name _____   **Date** _____

Preparation Method _____

_____
_____
_____
_____
_____
_____
_____
_____
_____
_____
_____
_____

Did you like this fruit?

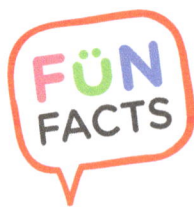 Rambutan are closely related to lychee fruit. However, it is easy to tell the two apart. Rambutan have red skin with soft, neon green, hairs all around them.

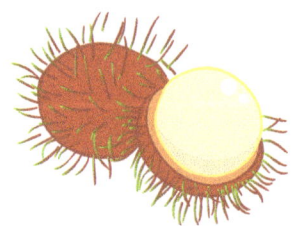

Pretend you're a chef! Create a fruit salad recipe:

Name Your Salad

List Your Ingredients

Describe Your Preparation Method

Fruit Name _____   **Date** _____

Preparation Method _____

_____

_____

_____

_____

_____

_____

_____

_____

Did you like this fruit?

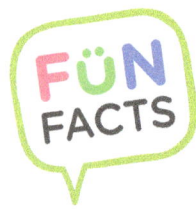 The common name for tamarillos in its native Andean region is "sachatomates" meaning "false tomato" because of their resemblance to tomatoes.

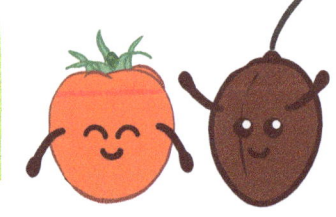

Fruit Name _____ **Date** _____

Preparation Method _____

Did you like this fruit?

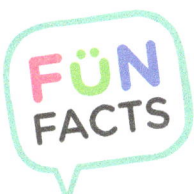 Baked breadfruit smells similar to fresh-baked bread! This is how breadfruit got its name.

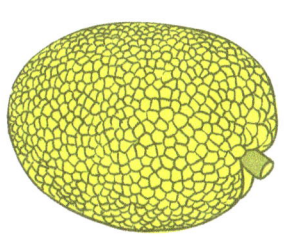

Fruit Name _____ **Date** _____

Preparation Method _____

Did you like this fruit?

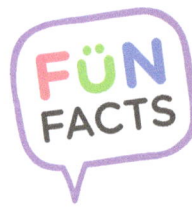

Blackberries are not true berries. True berries form from a flower with a single ovary and blackberries form from a flower with several ovaries that come together and form an aggregate fruit.

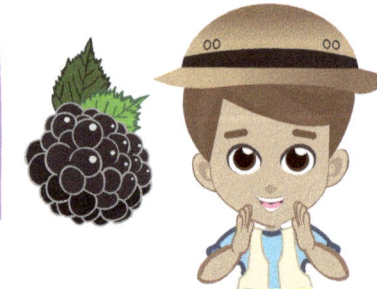

Fruit Name _____   **Date** _____

Preparation Method _____

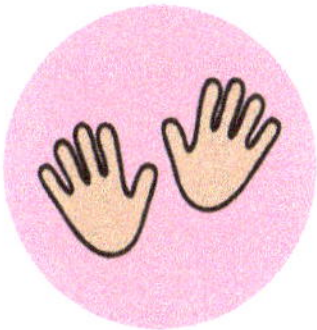

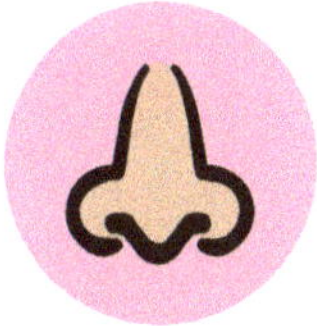

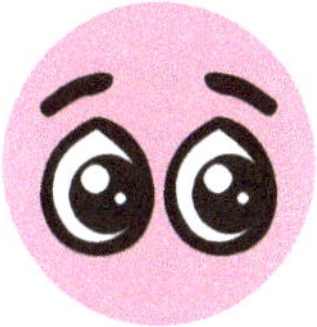

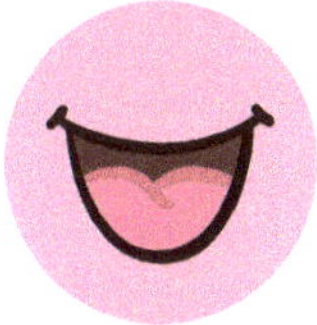

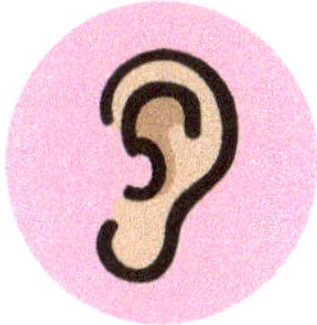

_____

_____

_____

_____

_____

Did you like this fruit?

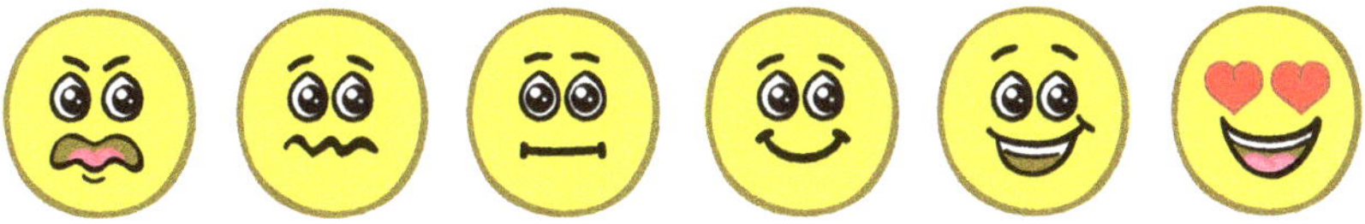

Draw what you're tasting!

Fruit Name _____   **Date** _____

Preparation Method _____

_____

_____

_____

_____

_____

Did you like this fruit?

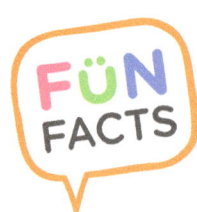 Unripe papayas are often eaten as a vegetable in savory dishes. Have you ever tried an unripe papaya?

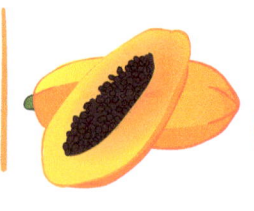

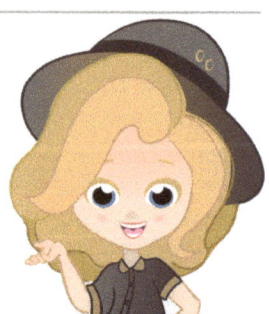

Let's try fruit varieties!

Fruit Name _____

Draw the variety and describe its flavor using descriptive words.

Variety: **Variety:** **Variety:**

Fruit Name _____

Draw the variety and describe its flavor using descriptive words.

Variety: **Variety:** **Variety:**

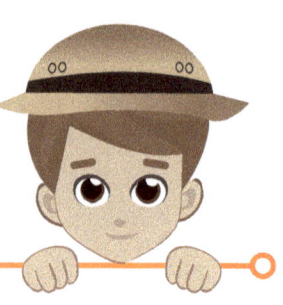

What did you discover by using this fruit journal?

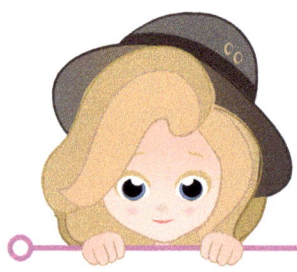

How did you decide whether or not you liked a fruit?

Are there any textures you loved or disliked?

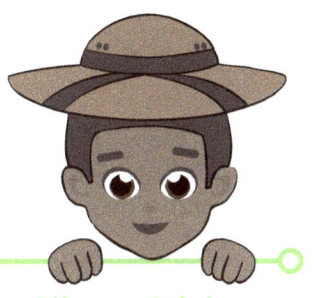

Buttery · Chewy · Fibrous · Juicy · Mushy · Slimy · Sticky

Continue your adventures in fruit and print additional "My 5 Senses Worksheets" from the Freebies tab on our website (www.experiencedeliciousnow.com)

www.ingramcontent.com/pod-product-compliance
Lightning Source LLC
Chambersburg PA
CBHW041319110526
44591CB00021B/2842